CW00704906

Dr. SEB

The Truth behind Liver Detox: Cleanse your body, find the Secret Natural way to improve your Health

AMBER FLOREY

© Copyright 2021 - All rights reserved.

The content contained within this book may not be reproduced, duplicated or transmitted without direct written permission from the author or the publisher.

Under no circumstances will any blame or legal responsibility be held against the publisher, or author, for any damages, reparation, or monetary loss due to the information contained within this book; either directly or indirectly.

Legal Notice:

This book is copyright protected. This book is only for personal use. You cannot amend, distribute, sell, use, quote or paraphrase any part, or the content within this book, without the consent of the author or publisher.

Disclaimer Notice:

Please note the information contained within this document is for educational and entertainment purposes only. All effort has been executed to present accurate, up to date, and reliable, complete information. No warranties of any kind are declared or implied. Readers acknowledge that the author is not engaging in the rendering of legal, financial, medical or professional advice. Dr.Sebi is not a doctor and before any attempts to use any of this information you should consult with your physician first.

Table of Contents

CHAPTER 5: 9 STEPS TO A FULL BODY DETOX

CHAPTER 6: HOW TO NATURALLY REVERSE DIABETES AND LOWER YOUR BLOOD PRESSURE

Introduction

In this industrialized society, chemicals are commonly found in the air we breathe, in the food we consume and in everyday household items like cleaners and cosmetics. These chemicals have many harmful effects; the principal is that they accumulate in our system and also prevent us from losing weight.

Obesity is a severe problem affecting a large part of the urban population. While many factors contribute to this, research has revealed that the environment's chemicals play a vital role in this.

How toxins in your body can be detrimental to your health

As per the latest data, 2 out of 3 adults living in the USA suffer from obesity. Obesity could lead to severe health conditions like diabetes, stroke, cancer, and heart disease. The good news is that by losing a small percentage of your weight, you can enhance your self-confidence, along with blood sugar, cholesterol, and blood pressure.

When your body is healthy, it can optimally detoxify itself, but sometimes your body's defence measures can be overwhelmed by prescription drugs, toxic air, and contaminated food. The liver's ability to detoxify weakens when there is a build-up of toxins present in our body.

Certain toxic substances linger inside our bodies. Our systems cannot flush them out efficiently, hampering our natural metabolism and leading to various disorders characterized by puffiness, bloating, and fluid retention.

Take diabetes, for example. In the United States, diabetes causes too many deaths each year. Research reveals that an individual is more likely to get diabetes if exposed to environmental toxins like dioxin and arsenic.

Arsenic is a natural element commonly found in the earth's crust, with the concentration being 1.5-3 mg/kg. This element is majorly transported via water; however, it is present in the air in urban settings in the United States at 0.02 $\mu g/m3$ and the water at an average of 0.0001 ppm.

Inorganic arsenic is formed when it is fixed with elements such as sulphur, chlorine, and oxygen. Arsenic takes an organic form in living organisms by reacting with hydrogen and carbon, but this form is significantly less harmful than inorganic arsenic.

The general population is exposed to arsenic, mainly through drinking water with a high chemical concentration. Water stored in wells often contains high levels of arsenic, and as per estimations, around 350,000 individuals in the USA consume arsenic-contaminated water regularly.

However, water is not the only source through which arsenic can enter our bodies. Individuals who work in specific fields may be exposed to the chemical, which can be found in medicines. Diseases like bronchial asthma, psoriasis, and leukaemia are often treated with drugs that have a high concentration of arsenic.

Even mineral water and wine have some arsenic present in them, and in the case of wine, the contamination occurs through the use of pesticides that contain the chemical. Many food items also contain organic and inorganic arsenic in varying amounts.

Sea-food, especially, is high in arsenic, and it could constitute more than 50% of the net daily arsenic intake. However, this is primarily dependent on the diet, followed by the population. Individuals working in lead, gold, and copper mines have a high chance of being exposed to arsenic. It is also used in dyes, pigments, pharmaceutical products, and glass.

Unlike arsenic, dioxin enters our bodies mainly through the food we consume. It is a fat-soluble substance, so it can be found in high concentrations in animal-based food like eggs, fish, pork, chicken, milk, and beef.

Dioxin persists in the environment for a long time, and its most deadly form is known as TCDD. Despite it mot being a naturally occurring substance, and industries are conducting large-scale manufacturing of dioxin, paper mills often produce this substance while carrying out the chlorine bleaching procedure.

Furthermore, water treatment plants produce dioxin during chlorination, and a few organic chemicals can be contaminated with this substance during the manufacturing process. Nevertheless, dioxide is spread in the environment mainly via incinerators burning chlorinated waste products.

Many people working in public health departments are concerned about the presence of dioxin in our environment and food. Several studies have been carried out to assess the toxic effects of TCDD. The animals used in these experiments have displayed immunotoxicity, carcinogenicity, weight loss, neurotoxicity, hepatotoxicity, and reproductive toxicity.

Although some studies have been conducted on humans as well, the results are somewhat inconclusive. When exposed to TCDD, humans show skin diseases, excess hair, pigment discoloration, etc. In some cases, it has been found that TCDD damages the liver and affects the urine and blood. It may also lead to hormonal and metabolical changes.

A Proposed Solution

Dr.Sebi, a renowned Honduran herbalist, advised his followers to avoid dead, hybrid, and genetically modified food, as well as drugs, in order to cleanse their organs. He believed that organically grown vegetables and fruits could fight the acidic waste material present in our bodies. Following this recommended diet is a bit difficult if you're a person who likes eating out. Thus, it requires you to cook most of your food at home.

Dr.Sebi helped many people deal with their health problems while he was alive. Although he is no more, his knowledge of detoxification and his healing techniques for hypertension and diabetes inspires people to this date. Some diseases like hypertension and diabetes have no definite cure in allopathic medicine, leading people to look for alternative treatment options.

While some people starting with a plant-based diet look to be fully cured, others follow it to alleviate prescription drugs' harmful side effects. Millions of people worldwide suffer from high blood pressure and diabetes, but most of them go for treatment rather than cure their ailments. However, you should be aware that it is possible to fix them by following an alkaline diet.

Chapter 1

Alkaline plant-based diet

B efore we get into detoxification and cleansing details, we need to understand what an alkaline plant-based diet is.

What is the alkaline diet?

It has been said that an alkaline diet is based on the concept that your diet influences the pH value of your body; alternatively, this diet is also known as an alkaline ash diet or acid-alkaline diet. The pH value indicates whether your body is acidic or alkaline. When food is consumed, it is broken down into usable energy via a process known as metabolism. It is similar to a fire that disintegrates solid material and is based on a chemical reaction.

However, this chemical reaction is a slow and gradual process, and like all reactions, it leaves behind some residue. When fire burns a matter, it leaves behind ash, and when food is broken down, it leaves behind metabolic waste, which can be acidic, alkaline, or neutral in nature. Advocates of an alkaline diet claim that the acidity of your body is directly influenced by metabolic waste.

Hence, upon consuming food that produces acidic residue, your blood also turns acidic. Conversely, your blood turns alkaline when you consume food that leaves an alkaline residue. There is a hypothesis, which states that acidic residue increases the chances of getting a disease, while alkaline ash protects your body against illnesses.

Thus, if your diet includes alkaline food, you can turn your body alkaline as well, improving your well-being. Sulphur, phosphate, and protein are some of the food components that leave an acidic residue, while potassium, magnesium, and calcium are alkaline components.

In order to maintain good health, you must make sure your blood has a constant pH. If the pH were to fluctuate frequently and exceed the normal range, the cells in your body would cease functioning, leading to severe complications. If you do not receive immediate treatment in such a situation, you might perish swiftly.

Fortunately, our bodies have several measures in place that allow them to maintain the pH balance. When your body is healthy, the pH of blood will likely be significantly altered by food. However, tiny changes in the pH level are quite common, and food can also affect your urine's pH level. If there is excess acid in your body, it is removed through the urine.

For instance, if you consume a large amount of meat, acid can be found in your urine for many hours since it takes some time for your body to get rid of all the metabolic waste. Thus, it is clear that we cannot determine the entire body's pH just by finding out the pH of urine. Besides, there are other factors that determine the pH of urine.

You can use pH strips to test your body's pH level. These strips are easy to use, and you can use them at home to calculate your body's pH quickly. If your urine's pH lies between 6 - 6.5 in the morning and between 6.5 - 7 in the evening, you know there is nothing to worry about. You can also use the strip to check your saliva's pH, and if it remains between 6.5 and 7.5 throughout the day, you know your body is functioning as expected. The testing is best conducted one hour prior to a meal or two hours after eating.

By testing your urine, you can get an indication of how efficiently your body is getting rid of acid and minerals like potassium, sodium, magnesium, calcium, etc. These are buffer minerals that protect the body from excess alkalinity or excess acidity. That being said, even when the optimum level for buffer minerals is maintained, the body can still turn excessively acidic or alkaline.

When the body produces too much alkali or acid, it must be expelled. This is usually done through urine. If the pH of urine is less than 6.5, it means that the buffer system is no longer working. You should immediately pay attention to declining acid levels to alleviate the autotoxication condition.

When it comes to blood, the pH should remain strictly between 7.36 and 7.44. If you are following a diet that's rich in animal protein, caffeine, sugar, etc., it becomes difficult for the body to regulate the internal systems and maintain balance. Thus, the body attempts to provide excessive buffering that can lead to the depletion of minerals like calcium, magnesium, potassium, and sodium making it more likely for you to suffer from degenerative diseases.

When the body is highly acidic, minerals are often extracted from bones and organs to neutralize the acid and get rid of it safely. This puts a lot of strain on the body and causes prolonged damage that might not be easy to detect. For this reason, you can follow an alkaline diet if you wish to detox your body.

What to eat and avoid

People following the alkaline diet are advised to consume more alkaline food and avoid acidic food. As per the rules of this diet, all food can be divided into acidic, neutral, and alkaline categories.

- Acidic food: Alcohol, eggs, dairy, fish, meat
- Neutral food: Sugar, starch, natural fat
- Alkaline food: Vegetables, legumes, nuts, fruits

When you follow the alkaline diet, you don't need to restrict your meals to certain hours or fast for long periods. Unlike other diets, this one does not tell you to eat certain foods and avoid others; instead, it advises people to follow a balanced diet by maintaining the acid-base continuum. Some of the foods recommended by this diet include:

- Lime juice
- Lemons
- White and red wine
- Coffee
- Vegetables
- Fruits

Some of the acid-producing foods that are not recommended by the alkaline diet are:

- Legumes
- Grains
- Eggs
- Dairy
- Fish
- Poultry
- Meat

This diet encourages you to eat more vegetables and fruits while cutting down on soda or totally removing it from your diet. You are also advised to drink around 64 ounces of mineral water every day and add lemon to water to alkalize your body. You should also reduce the amount of animal protein you consume daily and swap carbohydrates like rice or spaghetti with vegetables. Some people are also known to prepare an alkaline broth using vegetables.

Health benefits

Let us take a look at the various health benefits of the alkaline diet.

Bone Structure Maintenance and Development

The minerals you consume help maintain and develop your body's bone structure. Research has revealed that including alkalizing vegetables and fruits in your diet protects you from degenerative bone and muscle diseases.

An alkaline diet is beneficial for your bones because it helps your body achieve a balance of essential minerals that help in bone development and maintain muscle mass. Some of these minerals are phosphate, magnesium, and calcium. This diet also allows for better absorption of vitamin D and enhances growth hormone production.

Reduces Risk for Stroke and Hypertension

An alkaline diet enhances growth hormone production and reduces inflammation, thus slowing down the ageing process. Therefore, your cardiovascular health is improved, and you are protected against conditions like memory loss, stroke, kidney stones, hypertension, and high cholesterol.

Alleviates Inflammation

Chronic acidosis is a major contributing factor or joint pain, inflammation, menstrual issues, muscle spasms, headaches, and back pain. An alkaline diet, when followed on a regular basis, can reduce inflammation and chronic pain conditions.

Improves Vitamin Absorption and Wards Off Magnesium Deficiency

Magnesium is an essential mineral required for the proper functioning of bodily processes and enzymes. People suffering from magnesium deficiency often experience heart trouble, anxiety, insomnia, headaches, and muscle pains. Magnesium is also used to activate vitamin D, which is essential for the proper functioning of the endocrine and immune systems. An alkaline diet can provide you with the magnesium your body needs.

Boosts The Immune System and Protects Against Cancer

When there aren't enough minerals present in the body's cells, it cannot oxygenate the body or eliminate the waste. The body starts losing minerals to make up for vitamin absorption, as toxic substances accumulate inside your system and turns the immune system weak.

It is not yet proven that an alkaline diet can prevent cancer. However, there is some research to back up the fact that cancerous cells are more likely to die inside a body that's alkaline. When your body's pH becomes alkaline, some changes occur in the electric charges, and a few essential components are released from proteins. By reducing inflammation, an alkaline diet can also reduce the likelihood of cancer.

Who is the alkaline diet best for?

In reality, everyone could reap the advantages of an alkaline diet. If you are suffering from heart-related ailments, you can benefit from an alkaline diet. In this diet, you will be having more fruits and vegetables instead of foods rich in calories and fat. You will also avoid processed foods that contain a high amount of sodium. All of this reduces cholesterol and blood pressure, which are the major contributing factors to heart disease.

If you are overweight, you should consider following an alkaline diet. Since this type of diet does not include animal proteins and fats, you will find it easier to lose weight. This will help you prevent diseases like osteoarthritis and diabetes.

There are certain studies that show that chemotherapy drugs work more efficiently in an alkaline environment. While this does not essentially mean that cancer patients should follow an alkaline diet, you can always discuss this with your doctor.

Chapter 2

Disease reversal with detoxification and cleansing

Now, let us discuss in detail how disease reversal is possible through detoxification and cleansing.

How does detox help prevent potential diseases?

You must have heard all the fuss about "detox" and cleansing your body. There are several misconceptions when it comes to detoxification diets because your body has its own detox mechanism. In order to clear these out, we need to understand how detox works.

The detoxification process occurs inside the body and utilizes vital nutrients that you get from the food and drinks you consume. In this process, toxins are transformed into less harmful substances so they can be easily expelled from your body. You can categorize these toxins into two main groups: toxins produced by the body during the metabolism and those coming from external sources like food, air, and drinks.

Your body produces toxic substances like area, lactic acid, and other waste material generated by gut bacteria. Toxins coming from external sources include seafood rich in mercury, tobacco laced with chemicals, alcohol, drugs, and polluted air.

The detoxification process also involves the metabolization and removal of medications from your system. Toxic substances are harmful to your body, and they must undergo a transformation and be removed through sweat, respiration, faeces, and urine. Your body's ability to detoxify itself depends on factors like your diet, the environment you live in, genetic factors, and the lifestyle you follow. Thus, some individuals may require additional detoxification to support their body's natural cleansing process.

Sometimes the number of waste materials in your body can be much more significant than what your body can remove. In that case, they may accumulate in the bones, soft tissues, and fat cells, thus adversely affecting your health. This is the reason why additional detox mechanism may be needed in some instances.

The majority of detox programs require you to give up on processed food and those that produce the most toxins, like red meat, peanuts, eggs, gluten, and dairy. These programs also advise you to consume naturally grown fruits and vegetables, lean protein, seeds, nuts, and gluten-free grains. Some might recommend intermittent fasting, but this can carry potential risks for some individuals, doing more harm than good by suppressing the body's natural detoxification process. For this reason, experts in the medical field often advise against fasting.

These days, many people with absolutely no credentials claim to be detoxification experts. You must remember that not all detoxification programs are backed by research. Additionally, some programs might be potentially hazardous for people with existing health conditions, those on medication, breastfeeding and pregnant women, and people with eating disorders.

Although there are many reasons why people choose detoxification, it is mostly about feeling better and leading a healthier life. While detoxification has various health benefits, the major one is that it allows you to prevent potential diseases. Bad bowel health is a common reason for many diseases. When your body's toxicity level is exceptionally high, your bowel health deteriorates. In that case, a detoxification program can bring you back to good health by excreting most of the toxins.

However, before choosing a detox program, you need to consider certain factors like eating habits and lifestyle. You should also pay attention to your current and past health condition. Although the human body is designed to support a healthy lifestyle, the modern industrial world exposes us to a lot of stress and fills out minds and bodies with toxic substances. Thus, a lot of pressure is put on the body to function normally.

Symptoms of a toxic liver

The liver is a vital part of the digestive system. It is responsible for cleaning out toxins from your blood, producing proteins for clotting your blood, storing glucose, helping in fat digestion, producing bile, and process medicines, among many other things. The organ is also quite forgiving and is capable of regenerating cells up to a certain extent. However, repeated damage can cause your liver to become toxic, scarred, or inflamed. A high intake of toxins or alcohol is one of the many reasons why your liver may become unhealthy.

Toxic liver, or toxic hepatitis, can be defined as inflammation of your liver due to the reaction to certain substances that you have ingested. It can be caused by consuming certain nutritional supplements, drugs, chemicals, and alcohol.

At times, toxicity in the liver may develop within a few hours or days of exposure to the toxin. Some may take months of daily use before the symptoms and signs start to appear.

In most cases, a toxic liver's symptoms will start disappearing once the exposure to the toxin stops. However, the condition can damage your liver permanently, leading to cirrhosis (permanent scarring of the liver tissue) and, in some cases, liver failure.

Mild forms of toxic hepatitis may not be enough to cause any symptoms and can only be detected in blood tests. Some signs of a toxic liver include:

- Dark-yellow colored urine
- Weight loss
- Fever
- Rash
- Vomiting and nausea
- Loss of appetite
- Fatigue
- Abdominal pain on the upper section of the abdomen
- Excess and constant itching
- Yellowing of the whites of the eyes (jaundice) and skin

If you notice any signs and symptoms that may worry you, it is important that you see a doctor immediately. Overdosing on some medication like acetaminophen (for example, Tylenol) can lead to liver damage. It is essential you get immediate help if a child or an adult accidentally overdose on acetaminophen. Some signs of an acetaminophen overdose include:

- Coma
- Upper abdominal pain
- Vomiting and nausea
- Loss of appetite

What are some causes of these symptoms of a toxic liver?

A toxic liver can occur when inflammation starts developing in your liver due to over-exposure to a toxic substance. The condition may also develop due to consuming excessive over-the-counter or subscription medication.

Typically, the liver will break down and remove most of the chemicals and drugs found in the bloodstream. This process creates by-products and can potentially damage the liver. While it is true that your liver can regenerate, constant exposure to the toxic substance can cause, sometimes irreversible, harm.

Some reasons why you may develop toxic liver include:

Alcohol

Heavy drinkers are most susceptible to developing a toxic liver. Years of heavy drinking can cause alcoholic hepatitis – and inflammation in the liver and eventually lead to liver failure and, subsequently, death.

Over-the-counter pain relievers

Non-prescription pain relievers like naproxen (Aleve), ibuprofen (Motrin IB, Advil), aspirin, and the acetaminophen as mentioned earlier can damage your liver, especially if you combine it with alcohol or take it more than needed.

Prescription medication

Some types of medications are known to cause some severe liver damage. These drugs also include statin likes that are normally used to treat conditions like high cholesterol levels. Then, there is a combination of different drugs like anabolic steroids, certain antivirals, ketoconazole, niacin (Niaspan), azathioprine (Imuran, Azasan), phenytoin (Phenytek, Dilantin), clavulanate (Augmentin), etc. The list is almost endless.

Supplements and herbs

Some herbs are considered dangerous for the liver, like ephedra, kava, comfrey, chaparral, cascara, black cohosh, aloe vera, etc. As for supplements, liver damage can occur in children if they are mistaken as candies or consumed in large doses.

Industrial chemicals

If you work in an environment surrounded by chemicals, you need to be very careful. There are common chemicals that can cause toxic liver like polychlorinated biphenyls (a group of industrial chemicals), vinyl chloride (a chemical used to make plastics), carbon tetrachloride (used in dry cleaning solvents), paraquat (used in herbicides), etc.

What are some risk factors that increase toxic liver?

There are some risk factors that will increase your chances of toxic hepatitis like:

Taking certain prescription drugs or over-the-counter medicines/pain relievers

If you keep consuming prescription drugs or over-the-counter pain relievers and medicines, it will only increase liver toxicity risk. This is especially true if you take several medications in a day, in more than the prescribed doses.

Having a previous liver disease

If you are already suffering from non-alcoholic fatty liver disease or cirrhosis, your liver will be more susceptible to the effects of the toxins.

Having hepatitis

Chronic infection with a hepatitis virus (any one of them) is very rare. However, if it is possible, then it will make your liver more vulnerable to toxins.

Ageing

As with everything else, ageing may also contribute to a toxic liver. Additionally, the older you get, the slower your liver becomes in breaking down harmful substances. This means that the toxins and the by-products stay in your body longer.

Consuming alcohol

Drinking alcohol is bad for health. Even more so when mixed it with certain herbal supplements or medications. This will only increase the risk of liver toxicity.

Being female

The female biology can metabolize certain types of toxins slower than men. Therefore, their livers are exposed to higher blood concentrations of non-healthy substances for a longer time. In short, it increases the risk of developing toxic hepatitis.

Working in certain industries

If you work in specific industries, like chemical factories, you will be at risk of developing toxic liver.

(FROM HERE)

How to detox for digestive issues?

There are a lot of methods that can help you cleanse your digestive system. Some of them that can be done at home include:

Water flush

Drinking water daily and staying hydrated will help regulate and clean your digestive system. If you want to clear your liver of toxins and cleanse your colon, experts recommend at least six or eight glasses of lukewarm water every day.

Alternatively, you can also start eating fruits and vegetables high in water content like celery, lettuce, tomatoes, and watermelons. Actually, there are many more types of foods that can help clean your liver and colon naturally.

Saltwater flush

A saltwater flush, or also known as saltwater cleanse or a master cleanse, is the method to help you cleanse your digestive system, colon and liver by bringing in a forced bowel movement. Salt is needed for several biochemical processes like water balance regulation, nerve stimulation, nutrient absorption, muscle contractions, cell wall stability, and thyroid gland function.

Saltwater flush ignites your body's mechanism of waste elimination and natural detoxification so that your digestive system comes back on track and will make you feel lighter.

This method has been used for more than a decade by people to facilitate digestion and cleansing. All you need to do is drink a glass of saltwater in the morning and you will soon have the urge to go to the bathroom.

High-fiber diet

Foods that are rich in fiber are low and fat, and calories and will fill you up more. They also reduce the risk of specific health problems. However, the nutrients are still overlooked by many. Some fiber-rich foods include seeds, nuts, grains, vegetables, fruits, and much more.

The fibers and cellulose inside these items will bulk up excess matters in the colon. It will also regulate overactive bowels and constipation. If you want to keep your liver and colon healthy, ensure you eat many foods that contain high fiber content. Additionally, these foods are also helpful for gut bacteria.

Juices and smoothies

Juices and smoothies are popular choices for cleaning the liver and the digestive tract. It is recommended that you drink different varieties of juices to improve your liver's health and maintain your palate as well.

Fruits and vegetables, as mentioned above, contain nutrients and fiber that is beneficial for your body. You can drink many different types of juices, like vegetable juice, lemon, juice, apple juice, etc. However, experts suggest that drinking smoothies are much better than juices because they hold much more fibre.

More resistant starches

Like fibre, resistant starch is generally found in plant-based foods like grains, green bananas, legumes, rice, and potatoes. By boosting the gut microflora, these items will promote a healthy colon and liver. Additionally, they will also reduce the risk of certain cancers.

However, you need to be careful when ingesting resistant starch because it is normally found in carbohydrates. Hence, look for low-carb sources. Even in small quantities, these foods are great for cleansing your liver.

Probiotics

Another great option to clean your liver is adding probiotics to your diet. Additionally, you will also boost your overall health. You can take probiotic supplements for additional probiotics. Some other sources of probiotics include fermented foods like pickles, yogurt, etc.

Probiotics add good bacteria to the gut and stop inflammation. Additionally, regularity is promoted, which is an essential aspect of good digestive health.

Herbal teas

Herbal tea is a great choice to improve the health of your liver, gut, and digestive system. Laxative herbs like slippery elm, marshmallow root, aloe Vera, and psyllium are great for conditions like constipation. However, it is vital that you talk with a doctor before attempting to use these herbs. Also, do not consume them in large quantities. Try drinking three cups of herbal teas three times a day. As for laxative teas, only drink one cup per day.

Chapter 3

Liver cleanse

It may seem that new diets are popping up every day, trying to convince us that their unique formula is the ultimate solution for detoxifying the body and losing weight.

These products claim to cleanse your system and boost your metabolism to clean your liver with minimum effort and quick results. However, the scientific community has managed to capture these false promises and calling out their dishonesty. So, how do we know what is real and what is false?

Is liver cleanse possible?

A variety of medical websites, health practitioners, and supplement companies argue that the liver collects toxins during the filtering process for assimilation. According to them, these toxins will start displaying a wide range of non-specific symptoms over time. Eventually, it will lead to serious diseases and may even increase the risk of cancer. However, they are not a lot of evidence to prove their theories.

But, exposure to chemicals can undoubtedly damage your liver. For instance, alcohol is one of the most well-known ways to ruin your liver function over time.

In most cases, a liver detox or cleanse involves the following steps:

- Cleansing the gut and colon via enemas
- Observing a juice fast
- Avoiding certain types of foods
- Eating foods that are healthy for the liver
- Taking supplements that will flush out toxins out of the liver

Yes, liver failure is quite a serious health problem. But there is no proof that dangerous toxins accumulate in seemingly healthy livers without any type of exposure to these chemicals.

Modern medical practitioners often argue that the liver does not need any type of cleansing and detoxing. In fact, they state that doing so may even be dangerous.

Liver cleanse: Real or fake?

The liver is the largest internal organ of your body and is responsible for more than 500 different body functions like neutralizing toxins and detoxifying your body.

Since the liver is a detoxification organ, most of us think that liver detoxification will help your body recover after all the heavy partying in the weekends, boost your metabolism so that you end up losing weight, or give your body a kick-start towards a healthy life. However, these are just some of the things that the so-called medical practitioners want you to believe.

A healthy liver is capable of detoxifying itself. On the other hand, a liver detox will not make an unhealthy liver better. A person suffering from a liver disease needs proper medical treatment and may even have to make the appropriate dietary or lifestyle changes. In truth, you will end up wasting your money or do more damage to your body than good.

When we are talking about reality, we are always surrounded by toxins. However, our bodies have in-built mechanisms to help defend against them naturally.

Yes, you can definitely do things to improve your overall health and support healthy liver function. For instance, supplements like milk thistle can possibly improve the health of your liver, according to some research. However, there is no certain evidence that supplements like these will cleanse your liver or even cure any liver conditions.

1. Myths about liver cleanse

Here are some common myths about liver detoxification that are not true:

It is necessary

You will find a lot of liver detoxification supplements and products at medical stores and over the internet. Sadly, most of these products have not been regulated by the FDA, let alone been tested in clinical trials.

From this, it should be clear that there is no absolute proof that liver detoxification and cleansing work at all. In fact, it could do more harm than good. Therefore, if you decide to use supplements, do so with extreme caution.

Instead of these supplements and products, you can use these ingredients instead:

Milk thistle

As mentioned above, milk thistle is a well-known liver detoxification supplement full of anti-inflammatory and antioxidant properties. These properties will help reduce inflammation in the liver and other parts of the human body.

Turmeric

Turmeric is an ingredient that is filled with health benefits. One of the most benefits of turmeric includes decreasing the pro-inflammatory molecules that contribute to developing and worsening different types of diseases. Additionally, it will also reduce the risk of liver problems.

Since turmeric is something that cannot be found easily, you can also take it in its supplement form. You can refer to the manufacturer's label for the supplement dosage.

Additionally, it is crucial that you research these supplements. Consult your doctor regarding the benefits and the potential risks they may offer before using.

1. It helps in weight loss

2. It protects against liver disease

3. It helps with any existing liver damage

It helps in weight loss. There is no actual proof that the liver helps in weight loss. Additionally, it has been found that certain types of cleansing diets may slow down the body's metabolic rate; this means the process of weight loss, for which you are observing the diet, is slowed down!

Many people have claimed that they have lost weight by doing a liver cleanse. Little do they know, it is just fluid loss. Once they start eating normally again, they will quickly regain the lost weight.

There are three important factors that determine how quickly you lose weight. They include:

Calorie intake

It is recommended that a calorie intake of 1,600 to 2,400 is necessary for adult females. As for males, the daily required calorie intake is 2,000 to 3,000 calories. Based on your individual health, your doctor can provide you with an estimated calorie range you require.

Calorie output

It is a good idea to engage in some form of exercise to burn calories and lose weight. Curbing your food habits will not go long-term. Burning calories will help your body eliminate the extra weight.

Diet quality

While calories are very important, you decide to lower your calorie intake by consuming processed junk food. However, you will still not be able to lose weight. Processed junk food is always poor quality edibles and does not provide much nutrition to your body. If you want to lose weight and keep up your liver's normal functioning, you need to choose high-quality foods instead.

Some of these food items include:

- Proteins like eggs, fish, and chicken
- Healthy fats like nuts and olive oil
- Unrefined whole grains
- Fruits
- Vegetables

Switching your diet to high-quality unprocessed food will help you lose a substantial amount of weight. This is because your body decreases the calorie intake naturally while increasing the number of beneficial compounds like minerals and vitamins.

It protects against liver disease

As of now, no evidence supports that a liver Detox will protect against various liver diseases. Over 100 different types of liver diseases exist, some of which include:

- Non-alcoholic-related liver disease
- Alcohol-related liver diseases
- Hepatitis A, B, and C

The top two major risk factors for liver disease are excessive alcohol consumption and/or having a family history of liver diseases. While there are not a lot of things you can do about changing genetic factors, you can instead focus on lifestyle changes that can protect your liver against diseases. Some tips include:

Limiting the intake of alcohol

If you did not know already, alcohol is one of the toxics that your liver has to deal with. When you consume alcohol in excessive amounts, it will cause damage to your liver. For men up to 65, the recommended amount is two drinks per day and one drink for women. Once crossing the age of 65, men also should revert to one drink per day.

Moderate consumption of alcohol is one of the most critical factors that can protect against liver diseases. Additionally, do not consume medications like acetaminophen within 24 hours of drinking alcohol.

Hepatitis vaccination

Hepatitis is one of the most common liver diseases that is caused by a virus. If you feel that you are at increased risk, you need to get the Hepatitis A and B vaccinations; thankfully, there is also a treatment for Hepatitis C. But, all three are very dangerous to the liver. A good course of action is to protect yourself against exposure to these diseases.

Choose your medications carefully.

Your liver also processes medicines. Whether it is non-prescription or prescription drugs, you need to choose them carefully. If possible, speak to your doctor for alternatives. Also, you should never consume medications with alcohol.

Staying clear of needles

Hepatitis viruses are carried around the body via the blood. Hence, you should avoid sharing needles to inject medications or drugs. If you plan on getting a tattoo, always look for a shop that practices cleanliness and safety practices and is inspected and approved by the state's health department.

Maintain a healthy weight

As mentioned above, some non-alcohol-related issues can lead to liver diseases. Most of them are related to metabolic problems like Type-2 diabetes and obesity. The risk of liver diseases caused by these factors can be avoided simply by making healthy lifestyle choices.

Handle chemicals safely

Toxins and chemicals can gain entry into your body via the skin. Hence, it is important that you protect yourself by wearing long-sleeved shirts and pants, gloves, and masks when handling chemicals like paint, fungicides, and insecticides.

It helps with any existing liver damage.

There is no proof that a liver Detox can treat existing liver damage. However, it is a fact that some repairs are possible. When you damage your skin or other parts of your body, you develop a scar. However, your liver will generate damaged tissues by regenerating new cells, which makes it a unique organ.

However, this regeneration takes time. If you continue to damage your liver via poor diet, excessive consumption of alcohol, or drugs, it can hamper the regeneration process. Eventually, this will lead to liver scarring, which is irreversible. A severe level of scarring is known as cirrhosis.

Chapter 4

24 superfoods for natural liver detoxification

I t is very important that you take care of your liver. It is an important organ of the body and neglect will cause major liver-related problems. Some superfoods that help in natural liver detox include:

Lemon

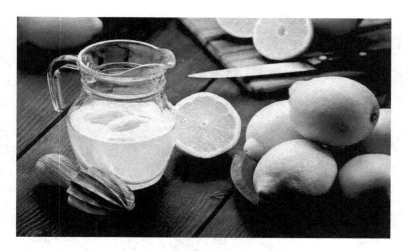

Lemons are a staple of different types of diets, especially the ones that focus on liver detox. One of the reasons for this is that lemons are packed with Vitamin C (a known antioxidant), which is perfect for fighting free radicals and for the skin. Additionally, lemons also have an alkaline effect on the body, which aids in restoring the natural pH balance and benefits the immune system as well.

You can start your day by filling a pitcher with some water, ice, and squeezed lemons. Apart from Vitamin C, lemon water will also provide a supply of copper, magnesium, and potassium. Your body also becomes more capable of absorbing more nutrients like calcium and iron from the other foods you eat. According to experts, better nutrient absorption leads to less bloating.

Lemon will also stimulate the liver and aid in flushing out the toxins because it acts as a mild diuretic. They also boost the production of liver detoxifying enzymes. In turn, you will be able to shed excess water weight as well.

Ginger

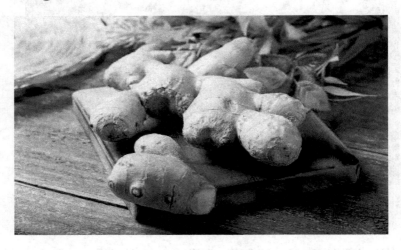

Ginger is a popular ingredient in the world of culinary and is also commonly used for treating various health conditions, including liver diseases. According to studies, it has been proven that people that consumed ginger daily had lower C-reactive protein (CRP, inflammatory marker), fasting blood sugar, LDL (bad) cholesterol, and ALT.

Ginger is rich in zinc, iron, manganese, copper, phosphorus, magnesium, riboflavin, niacin, and Vitamin B6. Metabolic and chemical analyses have revealed that ginger contains hundreds of metabolites and compounds. In fact, the oil resin from the roots of ginger, also known as oleoresin, contains many bioactive components.

Ginger roots contain powerful compounds like shoagaols and gingerols that protect against cellular damage and inhibit inflammation. Experts have concluded that the compounds show exert a variety of remarkable physiological and pharmacological activities. These compounds also support liver health and protect it against toxins like alcohol.

Generally, ginger is considered safe, even for people with existing liver conditions. However, it is always better if you consult with your healthcare provider before consuming high-dose ginger products.

Garlic and onion

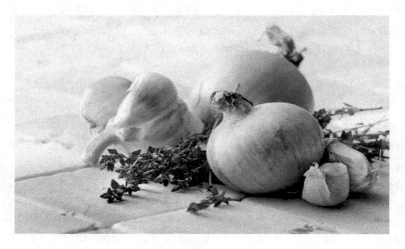

Garlic is a popular vegetable that is used for many herbal remedies. It is packed with potent antioxidant and anti-inflammatory plant compounds like ajoene, allicin, allicin, etc. that support the functioning of a healthy liver.

It has been studied by scientist that people that consumed garlic experienced significant reductions in triglyceride, LDL (bad) cholesterol, AST, and ALT levels. Additionally, these people also showed improvements in the severity of liver fat accumulation. Raw garlic has also been known to reduce the risk of liver cancer.

Similar to garlic, onions also contain allicin that flushes out the digestive tract and the liver. They also contain flavonoids, phytonutrients, fiber, and potassium to help your body do everything ranging from repelling toxic chemicals to fighting a nasty cold. While they may not smell so great, they are known to be one of the best foods for detoxifying the liver.

However, do not eat a lot of raw onions as it can lead to possible indigestion.

Grapefruit

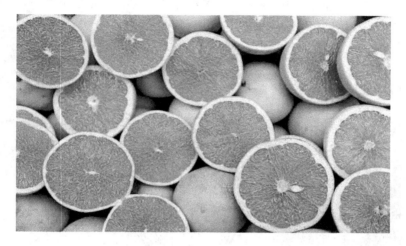

Grapefruit is another great choice for liver detoxification. It contains antioxidants that protect the liver naturally. The two main antioxidants found in grapefruit are naringin and naringenin. A lot of studies and research by experts have to lead to the conclusion that these compounds will help protect the liver from any injury.

The protective nature of grapefruit is known to occur in any one of two ways - by protecting cells and reducing inflammation. According to research, it has been shown that these antioxidants can reduce the development of hepatic fibrosis, which is a harmful condition that leads to excessive connective tissue build-up in the liver. This condition mostly happens due to inflammation.

Naringenin will decrease the number of fats in the liver and increase the production of enzymes that will be required to burn the fat. This prevents the excess fat from accumulating. Naringin will also improve the ability to metabolize alcohol and negate some of its effects. Hence, it can be concluded that eating grapefruit is a good way to maintain the health of your liver by fighting inflammation and damage.

Green grasses

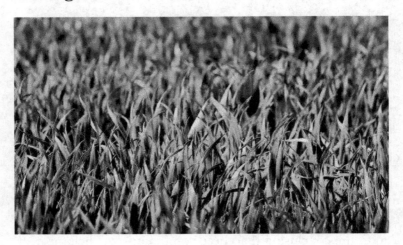

Green grass is a superfood that will provide you with a wide range of benefits. It is mostly consumed in the form of fresh juice; however, it can also be taken in powdered form. Since it is a superfood, green grass is packed with different nutrients that make it useful for the body. It is filled with therapeutic benefits and is known as complete nourishment.

Green grass contains proteins, chlorophyll, Vitamins (B Complex, K, E, C, A), amino acids, phytonutrients, magnesium, enzymes, calcium, and iron. The chlorophyll will eliminate stored toxins and impurities and support the healthy functioning of the liver. Once your body gets cleansed, you will notice better overall health as well as an increase in energy levels.

Green grass also has high levels of enzymes that aid in digestion. They break down the food so that it becomes easier to absorb the nutrients. Green glass also has detox effects that will clean your liver and intestines so that you experience abdominal discomfort, bloating and less gas.

Artichoke

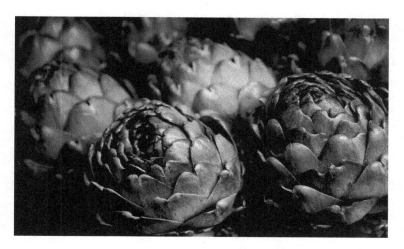

Artichokes are a type of vegetable that has been used for medicinal uses for centuries. It is packed with powerful nutrients like protein, fiber, fat, Vitamins (B6, C, K), iron, calcium, zinc, etc. Artichokes are also low in fat and particularly high in folate.

Artichoke leaf extract can protect your liver from damage and also promotes the growth of new tissue. It also promotes the production of bile, which will remove harmful toxins from your liver. It also has been studied that artichoke extract results in better liver function, higher antioxidant levels, and less liver damage.

It has also been concluded that artichoke extract also prevents non-alcoholic fatty liver disease, which results in a less fat deposition as well as reduced liver inflammation. According to scientists, certain antioxidants found in artichokes – silymarin and cynarin – are partly responsible for these benefits.

Overall, consuming artichokes daily will protect your liver against damage and aid in relieving non-alcoholic fatty liver disease. Many studies are being done on the benefits of artichokes.

Citrus fruits

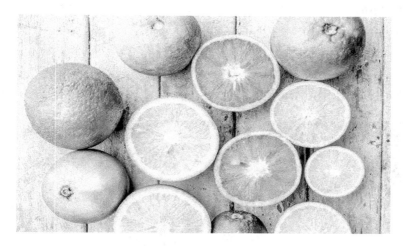

Citrus fruits like oranges have been used as food and traditional treatment for scurvy, the deficiency of Vitamin C. While the benefits of citrus fruits have been recognized for centuries, its specific mechanisms of action are still yet to be determined. Hence, various research laboratories are actively engaged in studying the components of citrus fruits. With that being said, recent medical reports have concluded that citrus fruits contain a plant pigment known as cryptoxanthin, which improves the health of your liver significantly.

It has been studied that citrus fruit extract will increase the levels of cryptoxanthin in the liver, kidney, and spleen. This pigment is also detected in the blood, which only suggests that it offers long-term benefits to the liver and other organs of your body.

For the liver, exposure to cryptoxanthin will lower the risk of developing liver diseases. Additionally, citrus fruits are also known to lower the risk of problems related to liver function that is caused by the consumption of alcohol. Citrus fruits will improve the cellular activities in your liver and protect against various types of diseases.

Seaweed and ocean salt

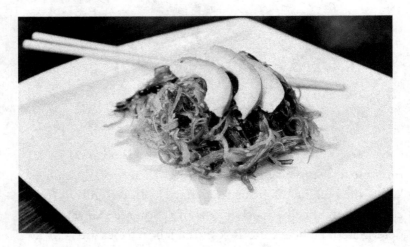

Seaweed and ocean salt are derivatives of salty water. Seaweeds are packed with nutrients that encourage the process of flushing toxins and support the overall health of the liver. Seaweeds are rich in minerals and iodine to promote a healthy metabolism. These nutrients stimulate the liver to remove toxins from the body. Additionally, it also promotes elimination through the skin, kidneys, and intestines. Seaweeds are also rich in antioxidants, anti-fungal, anti-parasitic, and anti-viral properties that help eliminate free radicals. This improves liver function by decreasing triglyceride and cholesterol levels.

The body's natural detoxification process can cause the pH of the blood to become more acidic. In this case, the minerals found in ocean salt can help buffer this condition. Additionally, toxins deplete minerals like magnesium that can lead to deficiencies of certain enzymes that help in the detoxification process of the liver. Ocean water is also known to accelerate the process of cell generation, especially those that are damaged by cirrhosis and other such conditions.

Beetroot

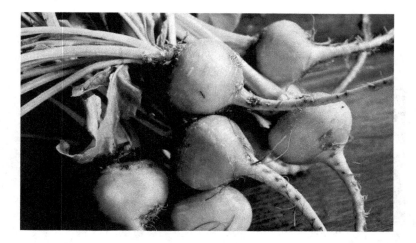

Recent research has found that fresh beetroot is a great choice for improving the health of your liver. It is an excellent liver cleanser, purifies the blood, and improves the overall circulation as well. Beetroot improves liver function by thinning the bile and allowing it to move more freely into the small intestine.

According to research, a high level of oxidative stress is liked directly to increased toxicity. The presence of betalain pigment in beetroot fights oxidative stress and removes free radicals that are associated with various disorders and diseases. Hence, antioxidants encourage the detoxification process and remove toxins from the body.

Beetroot also contains dietary fiber, which plays an important role in the detoxification process for organs like the kidneys, gut, and liver. It is important to flush toxins out of the body, and the dietary fibers present in beetroots help remove the toxins and encourage detoxification. Beetroot also contains glutathione to support the detoxification process and clearing out toxins from the body.

Green tea

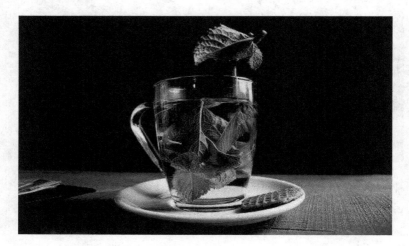

For overall well-being, green tea is considered one of the top beverages. With its foundations firmly rooted in traditional Indian and Chinese medicines, it contains a powerful combination of nutrients, trace minerals, and antioxidants. Apart from a refreshing drink, green tea is also an ideal supplement for exercising, detoxing, and cleansing.

The first step to detoxifying is eating wholesome, natural, and clean foods. Detoxing will help you feel more energized and less bloated while freeing your body from toxins. Antioxidant-rich green tea will naturally flush your system and help your body increase the production of detoxification properties.

While boosting your immune system, green tea will protect your liver from the damaging effects of substances like alcohol. Apart from helping detoxify your liver and your body, green tea will also improve your physical performance and increase fat burning, thereby boosting your metabolism. However, it is recommended to visit a doctor to understand how much green tea you should drink; this is because excess consumption of green tea can increase liver damage.

Cabbage

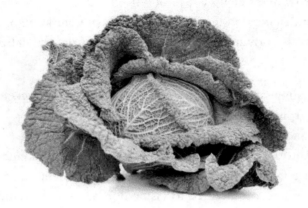

Cabbage is another healthy type of food that helps improve your liver conditions. Cabbage is a type of cruciferous vegetable, similar to broccoli, and is considered a liver-friendly food. It contains a high concentration of chemical compounds and phytonutrients that prove to be effective when it comes to helping the liver remove toxic substances from the blood.

Phytonutrients present in cabbages, according to research, have proven to remove harmful substances like metals, prescription and non-prescription drugs, chemicals, and pesticides that may get accumulated over time, and even carcinogens.

Cabbage is a healthy option for the body because it can lower the amount of cholesterol that is present in the body. Additional studies have proven to decrease the risk of many types of cardiovascular diseases. Cabbages also have diuretic properties that help get rid of excess toxins and liquid and clean your colon and liver.

Due to all these reasons, cabbage is commonly considered to be one of the healthiest vegetables you can find in the market.

Dark leafy greens

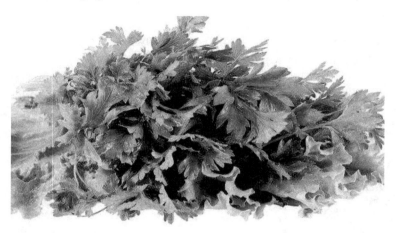

According to research in top institutions, nitrate compounds found in leafy green vegetables are capable of reversing and preventing liver fatty disease. Dark leafy greens like spinach and lettuce contain a high concentration of nitrate that fights against various liver problems, especially non-alcoholic fatty liver disease, a condition in which fats build up in the liver.

Fatty liver disease is one of the most common causes of chronic liver disease that is generally found in Western countries. Some primary causes of this health problem are excessive alcohol intake and a high-calorie and fatty diet.

Nitrates found in dark leafy greens are known to improve and boost cell metabolism. It is also suggested that some types of leafy greens also protect against certain metabolic conditions like Type-2 diabetes. Additionally, high consumption of vegetables and fruits will significantly improve cardiovascular function.

Various diseases of cardiovascular function, diabetes, and liver are connected. This connection is the nitrate levels that will decrease due to no physical activities, excessive drinking, and a fatty diet. Hence, eating leafy greens will increase the levels of nitrates present in your body.

Cruciferous vegetables

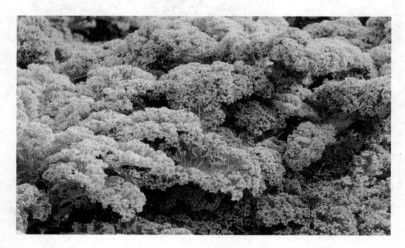

Cruciferous vegetables, or crucifers, include familiar vegetables like broccoli, cauliflower, cabbage (mentioned above), Brussels sprouts, and kale. Apart from imparting a delicious flavor to your food, they also possess a lot of health benefits like controlling inflammation, antioxidants, and detoxification. Through detoxification, these vegetables eliminate toxins from the body, thereby providing improved health, greater energy, and the power to prevent different types of illnesses like neurodegenerative disorders, auto-immunity, and cancers.

Cruciferous vegetables contain a lot of nutrients like fatty acids, antioxidants, minerals, and key vitamins. They also increase the levels of detoxification enzymes and protect the liver from potential damage. Apart from conventional nutrients, they also contain powerful compounds known as glucosinolates, which are potent detoxifiers. Cruciferous vegetables support both phases of detoxification. Additionally, these compounds are also potent antioxidants and reduce inflammation, which plays key roles in reducing the risk of autoimmune disease (like thyroid diseases, heart diseases, inflammatory disorders), prevent cancer, and support energy production.

Root vegetables

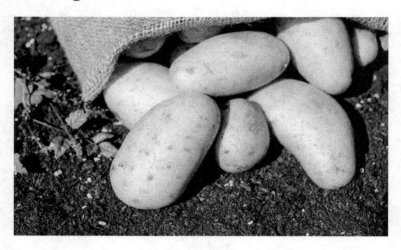

Different types of root vegetables like sweet potatoes, winter squash, chicory roots, and carrots are rich in beta-carotene, which is your body's favorite anti-inflammatory nutrient. Beta carotene converts Vitamin A in the body, directly in the liver. It is suggested that you get your dose of Vitamin A through beta carotene-rich foods instead of supplements.

Most supplements contain excess Vitamin A, which can be toxic for the liver; this is because Vitamin A gets stored more than excreted since it is a fat-soluble vitamin. However, root vegetables like sweet potatoes, which are rich in Vitamin A, do not cause any type of liver poisoning and are not stored for long-term use, unlike supplements.

Most root vegetables are also rich in Vitamin C, fiber, and many other immunity-boosting and cleansing nutrients that help in the normal functioning of your liver. You can roast these vegetables for a hearty dinner or create a simple lunch by stuffing them with some hummus and salsa for an easy lunch.

Fresh seasonal fruits

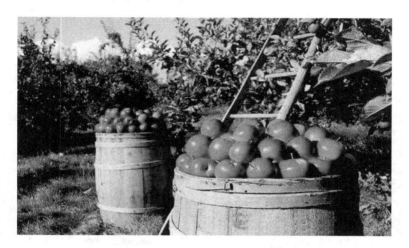

Seasonal fruits contain a lot of nutrients and antioxidants are connected to several health benefits. It has been studied that whole fruits, as well as the juices and extracts, will keep the liver healthy. Consuming fruits daily will protect the liver from damage. Additionally, it will also increase the production of antioxidant enzymes as well as increase immune cell response.

Additionally, it has been found that antioxidants found in most fruits commonly slow down the development of fibrosis and lesions, both of that lead to scar tissue in the liver. Further research states that these compounds also inhibit the growth of liver cancer cells; however, more studies are being done on this topic.

More studies have led to the conclusion that supplementing your diet with extracts of different fruits (like grapes) will improve the overall functioning of your liver.

Making fruits like apples, watermelons, and berries a regular part of your diet is one of the best ways to ensure that your liver is supplied with antioxidants so that your overall health remains in the best condition.

Nuts

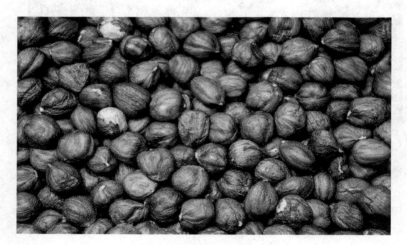

When it comes to the overall health of your body, nuts are not always shown in a positive light. This perception is mostly due to the popularity of nut products like honey-roasted snacks that are prepared with a lot of salt, sugar, and additional fats. However, if you eat nuts in their raw form, they are indeed a form of superfood. They are basically morsels filled with proteins and other nutrients. Since the liver requires additional nutrients, people will liver problems are advised to include nuts in their diets.

Nuts are one of the best natural foods for your liver – you will find a wide variety of them based on your taste and can be stored easily as well. Additionally, they have hard shells that protect them from environmental pollution and pesticides, they have a low risk of toxicity.

Nuts are extremely nutritious – they are a good source of protein, full of unsaturated and healthful fats, and high in antioxidants. Additionally, they also are good sources of other nutrients like Vitamin E, fiber, selenium, magnesium, niacin, and copper. Most nuts have a high concentration of amino acid arginine, which helps the liver detoxify ammonia.

Brown rice

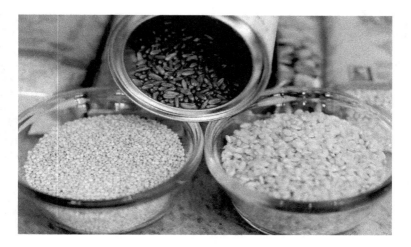

Rice has been a staple for the human diet for more than a thousand years. In fact, some rice farming tools were found in China that dates back more than 8,000 years ago. Today, there are roughly 40,000 varieties of rice grown. One of these is brown rice, which is considered the best type for liver health. Brown rice is whole grain; this is important because the less processed the grain, the more it is filled with nutrients.

The germ and bran, both outer layers of brown rice, contain most minerals and vitamins. These layers are removed when manufacturers make white rice, which is the reason why brown rice is a much healthier option.

Similar to other types of whole grains, brown rice is rich in Vitamin B, which will improve fat metabolism and liver function. These grains are lower in glycemic index and rich in filling fiber and minerals. Foods that are high in fiber lowers the storage of sugar in the liver, thereby avoiding the overload that can eventually lead to various liver complications.

Watercress

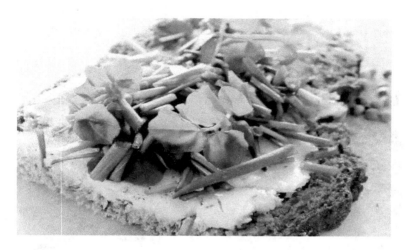

Watercress is a perennial vegetable that grows along running waterways. They also survive in various soil conditions, as long as the soils are saturated with water. Apart from its delicious flavor, watercress shoots and leaves have been used for medicinal purposes for a very long time. Watercress is related to other types of cruciferous vegetables like kale, cabbage, and broccoli.

As a cruciferous and leafy green vegetable, watercress is one of the top cancer-fighting foods. This is because it is rich in antioxidants, minerals, and vitamins. Additionally, it is low in sodium, carbs, fats, and calories.

Watercress also contains a lot of beneficial compounds. One of them is isothiocyanate, which occurs naturally in many cruciferous vegetables. It has been studied that the compound can effectively fight cancer-spreading cells and may even block their growth. Further studies have concluded that when broken down, these compounds also protect cells from DNA damage by inactivating carcinogens. This means that watercress can be used to fight other forms of cancer apart from liver cancer like breast cancer and lung cancer.

Turmeric

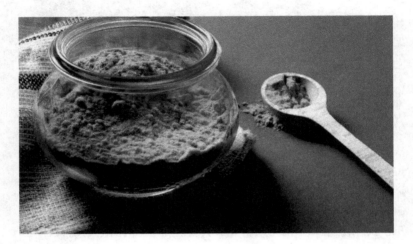

Turmeric has been used for many years for its potent medicinal properties. It contains 3-6% curcuminoids, which offer a wide array of health benefits. According to studies, curcumin has many healthy effects, thanks to its antifungal, antibacterial, and antiviral properties. Tests have proven that it can cure many inflammatory conditions like IBS (Irritable Bowel Syndrome), asthma, allergies, and even skin conditions like psoriasis.

Additionally, new research suggests that the antioxidant properties of curcumin promote liver health by acting as a detox agent in the body. In turn, this reduces the risk of various liver-related diseases. Curcumin also has shielding effects against other heavy metal toxicity like chromium, cadmium, arsenic, copper, and lead poisoning. The mechanisms of turmeric are enough to improve and repair liver health by free radical scavenging, stabilizing mitochondrial function, and maintaining antioxidant status.

As for cleansing and detoxifying the liver, turmeric will significantly reduce lipid peroxidase, which is the oxidative degradation of lipids; this way, it helps protect the liver from potential injury. Curcumin also suppresses hepatic oxidative stress, thanks to its therapeutic uses in the treatment and prevention of liver diseases.

Amla

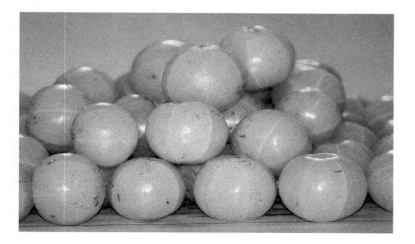

Amla, or Indian gooseberry, is good for liver health. It is loaded with all the essential nutrients that offer a lot of health benefits. It is regarded as the best source of Vitamin C. Additionally, the antioxidants present in it will clear the toxins from the body and protect the liver from damage.

Amla is also frequently used to treat problems like liver cirrhosis, people suffering from hepatitis, and in the rehabilitation of alcoholics with severe liver damage. Amla inhibits the onset of liver fibrosis, which is excessive liver inflammation caused by clinical conditions or liver injuries.

Amla juice is known to reduce cholesterol levels as the antioxidants and amino acids present in them aid in the overall functioning of the body. It also aids in flushing out toxins from the body and supports the normal working of the liver.

The wonderful fruit also acts as a natural remedy that prevents fatty liver disease. It is often used in various types of medications to exert liver-protection actions, along with digestive and immune-boosting action.

Green tea

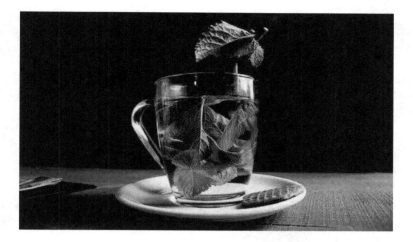

Green tea has been one of the most popular beverages for many years, thanks to the wide range of health benefits it offers. While it is mostly consumed for weight loss, green tea provides some other amazing health benefits as well.

According to research, a combination of exercise and green tea extract significantly reduces the severity of obesity-related fatty liver disease. It also reduces signs of non-alcoholic fatty liver disease, fight against oxidative stress, and reduces the overall fat content.

Green tea contains all the important antioxidants needed by the body, including catechins, which help protect the liver. It aids in the natural process of liver detoxification and also removes the potential risk from free radicals. Green tea also reduces the overall risk of other liver diseases like liver extent. The chances of Type-2 diabetes reduces, thereby lowering the risk for non-alcoholic fatty liver. Additionally, there is also a significant reduction in blood sugar levels and prevents the risk of diabetes.

Perhaps, the best aspect is that green tea is it can be consumed at any time of the day. However, you need to drink it in moderation. Excessive intake of green tea can lead to many harmful effects.

Avocado

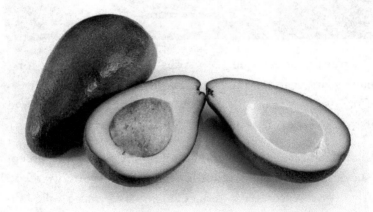

Eating avocado is an ideal choice for people with liver problems. While it is filled with many different kinds of health benefits, its antioxidant and anti-inflammatory properties and healthful fats make it a perfect food for a compromised liver.

Avocado is quite valuable for people with a fatty liver. Healthy fats improve the cholesterol profile by lowering the amount of low-density lipoproteins (LDLs) or also commonly known as bad cholesterol. Instead, it will raise the high-density lipoprotein (HDL), or good cholesterol.

Avocado helps the body produce glutathione, a type of antioxidant that protects the liver cells from damage and filter and removes harmful substances. People with chronic liver disease, mostly due to repeated injuries, often have low levels of glutathione. In such cases, consuming avocado is recommended.

Apart from glutathione, avocados are also rich in other nutrients like Vitamin E and C and filled with antioxidants that neutralize free radicals. Deactivating or neutralizing harmful free radicals is very important if you want to protect the liver cells from damage.

Walnuts

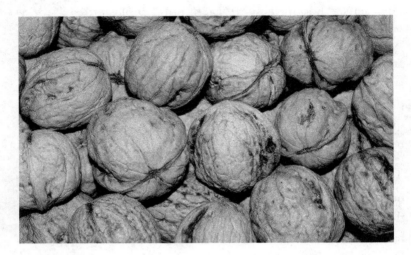

People that eat nuts every day are at a much lower risk of different serious diseases. Apart from being delicious, they are also convenient snacks. Hence, it is recommended that you include some walnuts in your diet each day.

According to studies, it has been found that people that eat walnuts every day are at lower risk of developing liver problems, heart diseases, etc. Since they are very tasty, including them in your diet is not a big problem. Sadly, this can also lead to allergies; hence, you should avoid them if you are prone to developing allergies.

Walnuts are very high in fiber content, which will keep you feeling sated. You will also gain a lot of other nutrients like essential fatty acids and other minerals like zinc, calcium, and magnesium. Walnuts contain omega-3 fatty acids, which are said to lower the fat levels in the liver. This makes them perfect for people with fatty liver disease.

The latest studies prove that eating walnuts will improve the liver function test results in people suffering from non-alcoholic fatty liver disease.

Olive oil

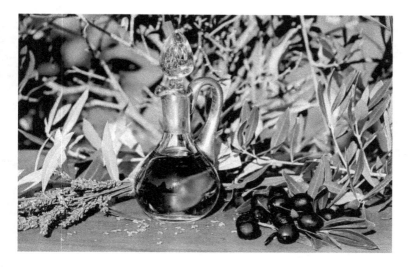

Olive oil is considered one of the best options for detoxifying your liver. It is considered a healthy fat that provides a lot of health benefits, including positive effects on metabolic health and the heart. It has been studied by experts that consuming one teaspoon of olive oil per day will improve fat levels and boost the production of liver enzymes.

Olive oil will also raise the level of a protein that is associated with positive metabolic effects. Additionally, you will also have a better flow to the liver and less fat accumulation. It has been studied that some effects of olive oil in your diet resulted in improved blood levels of the liver enzymes and improved insulin sensitivity.

Accumulation of fat in the liver is the first stage of any liver disease. Hence, the positive effects of olive oil on liver fats as well as other health aspects render it an important part of a diet. You can use this oil for cooking instead of conventional oils.

Chapter 5

9 steps to a full body detox

I t is often said that detox diets are designed to promote weight loss, improve health, and eliminate toxins from the body. Most of these diets contain foods that are thought to have detoxifying properties like teas, laxatives, etc.

However, the term 'toxin' is loosely defined in the context of detox diets. Toxins include processed foods, heavy metals, synthetic chemicals, pollutants, etc.; all these will negatively affect health. However, these diets rarely are able to identify specific toxins they aim to eliminate. Additionally, no evidence support using these diets for sustainable weight loss or toxin elimination.

The human body has a sophisticated way to eliminate toxins that involve the lungs, skin, digestive system, kidneys, and of course, the liver. But, these organs can only eliminate unwanted substances if they are healthy.

Overall, most detox diets do not do anything more than what your body cannot do naturally. However, they do optimize the natural detoxification system of the human body.

Common misconceptions

While detox diets may sound appealing, your body is more than capable enough to handle toxins and other unwanted substances.

Limit alcohol

Almost 90% of the alcohol you consume is metabolized in your liver. The enzymes released by your liver will metabolize alcohol to acetaldehyde, a chemical known to cause cancer. Since acetaldehyde is recognized as a toxin, your liver will convert it into acetate, which can then be eliminated from your body.

While there are some studies that show low-to-moderate consumption of alcohol is beneficial for your health, drinking over the recommended amount could cause a lot of health problems. Drinking more alcohol will severely damage your liver and cause scarring, inflammation, and a buildup of fat.

Once your liver starts developing these problems, it becomes unable to function adequately. Subsequently, it will not be able to do necessary tasks like filtering toxins and waste from your body.

In cases like these, one way to ensure that your body's detoxification system runs strong is to limit or even abstain entirely from alcohol.

According to health authorities, it is recommended to limit alcohol to two glasses (for men) and one glass (for women). In case you do not drink, you should not start since there are potential benefits associated with light-to-moderate consumption of alcohol.

Overall, drinking more alcohol than the recommended amount will reduce your liver's ability to carry out even normal functions, like detoxifying.

Get adequate sleep

It is extremely important that you get enough quality sleep each night; this will support your body's natural detoxification system as well as boost your overall health. Apart from eliminating toxic waste by-products that may get accumulated throughout the day, sleeping will also allow your brain to recharge and re-organize itself.

One of these toxic waste by-products includes a protein known as beta-amyloid, which plays an important role in the development of Alzheimer's disease. Not getting enough sleep will cause your body to not get the time to perform those functions. In due time, the toxins will start accumulating and affect different aspects of your health as well.

According to studies, it has been found that poor sleep will always have both short and long-term consequences, like obesity, Type-2 diabetes, heart diseases, high blood pressure, anxiety, and stress.

The amount of sleep you need to is roughly 6 to 9 hours every night if you want to promote good health. If you have difficulties falling and staying asleep, you can make certain lifestyle changes like limiting blue light that is emitted from computer screens and mobile devices before bedtime and/or sticking to a proper sleep schedule.

Once properly rested, your brain will recharge and reorganize itself, this will allow your body to eliminated toxins throughout the day.

Drink more water

Drinking lots of water is very important to maintain good health. Apart from the obvious task of quenching your thirst, water also aids nutrient absorption and digestion, lubricates the joints, regulates the body temperature, as well as detoxifies your body by eliminating waste products.

For the body to function optimally, the body's cells need to be repaired continuously so that they can effectively break down nutrients for your body to use as energy. On the other hand, while this process is important, it will also release waste in the form of carbon dioxide and urea; the buildup of these wastes can cause damage if they build up in your blood.

Water will transport carbon dioxide, urea, and other similar waste products and eliminate them from your body via sweating, breathing, and urination. Hence, it is crucial that you stay properly hydrated for optimal detoxification.

On average, it is recommended that you drink 3.7-liters (125-ounces) for men and 2.7-liters (91-ounces) for women. This amount can also vary on your activity level, your location, and your diet. Apart from its many roles in the human body, water will allow your body to detoxify and remove waste products from your blood.

Eat less sugar and processed foods

Today, processed foods and sugar are some of the most talked-about subjects when it comes to health. According to studies, consuming highly-processed and sugary foods has been linked to chronic diseases like diabetes, cancer, and heart diseases. Additionally, it has also been linked to obesity.

The diseases mentioned above will stop your body's natural ability to detoxify itself because it will harm the organs that play these important roles like kidneys and liver. For instance, consuming high amounts of sugary beverages can cause conditions like fatty liver, which will negatively impact the normal functioning of your liver.

You can keep your body's natural detoxification system healthy simply by cutting out junk food. The best way to limit junk food is to simply ignore and leave it on the store shelf. Having no junk food in your home will remove all temptations altogether.

Instead of storing junk food, you can replace them with healthier types of foods like vegetables and fruits. This is another way to reduce junk food consumption.

Junk food reduction will minimize your chances of developing chronic diseases like diabetes and obesity. It is quite crucial because these diseases can lead to serious health problems that will not allow you to detoxify your body efficiently.

Eat foods rich in antioxidants

Antioxidants are very important for the growth of your body. It protects the cells from free radicals, which causes significant damage to the body. Free radicals are excessively produced by a condition known as oxidative stress.

Naturally, your body produces these molecules for important cellular processes like digestion. However, habits like a poor diet, smoking tobacco, drinking alcohol, and exposure to pollutants can increase the production of excessive free radicals.

Free radicals can damage the cells of your body and are often responsible for a wide range of conditions like certain types of cancers, asthma, liver diseases, heart diseases, and dementia.

To help the body fight oxidative stress that can cause the production of excess free radicals and other toxins that will increase the risk of diseases, it is recommended by medical experts to eat a diet that is rich in antioxidants. But, it is important that you try getting as many antioxidants from foods and not supplements; if taken in large amounts, antioxidants from supplements can cause or increase the risk of certain diseases.

Some examples of antioxidants include zeaxanthin, selenium, Vitamin E, Vitamin C, and Vitamin A. Foods like spices, vegetables, cocoa, nuts, fruits, berries, and beverages like green tea and coffee have the highest amounts of antioxidants.

Eat foods high in prebiotics

The overall health of your gut is important, especially if you want to keep your detoxification system healthy. The intestinal cells have a detoxification and excretion system that will protect your body and hut from harmful toxins like chemicals.

Prebiotics is a type of fiber that feeds good bacteria present in your gut or also known as probiotics. Prebiotics are a precursor to good gut health. By feeding on prebiotics, the good bacteria produce short-chain fatty acids, a nutrient that is beneficial for your health.

However, certain conditions like diet quality, poor dental hygiene, or using antibiotics can disturb the balance between good and bad bacteria. As a result, this unhealthy shift will weaken your body's natural detoxification and immune systems, thereby increasing your risk of inflammation and disease.

Eating foods rich in prebiotics is important; they will keep your detoxification and immune systems healthy. Good food sources for prebiotics include oats, garlic, onions, asparagus, bananas, artichokes, and tomatoes. Eating these foods that are rich in prebiotics will keep your digestive system well and running, which is important to improve your immune health and proper detoxification.

Reduce your intake of salt

For some people, detoxification means eliminating excess water. Consuming more salt than is required will cause your body to start retaining excess fluid. This condition will end up affecting your liver or kidney – or even if you do not drink an adequate amount of water.

This excess buildup of fluid will start making you feel bloated and uncomfortable. If you find end up consuming too much salt, you can easily detoxify yourself from the excess water weight. One of the best ways to remove extra water weight (as a result of too much salt) is to increase your water intake.

When you increase your salt intake, your body will start releasing an antidiuretic hormone. This hormone will prevent you from urinating, which is a natural detoxification process.

While it may sound counterintuitive, drinking more water will help your body control and/or reduce the secretion of this antidiuretic hormone. It will also increase your urination, which will remove more waste products and water from your body.

You could also increase your consumption of the amount of foods that are rich in potassium. This will counterbalance some of the effects of sodium, which is present in salt. Some foods that are rich in potassium include spinach, bananas, kidney beans, squash, and potatoes.

Get active

Regardless of body weight, regular exercising is associated with a longer life and a reduced risk of many diseases and conditions like certain types of cancers, high blood pressure, heart diseases, and Type-2 diabetes.

Although there are many health benefits of physically working out, reducing inflammation is the most important one. While some types of inflammation are necessary for healing wounds and recovering from various infections, too much of it can end up weakening the natural immune system of your body and increasing the risk of diseases.

Exercising is the best solution for reducing inflammation. It will help your body's systems to work normally, including the detoxification process, and protect against different health problems.

Spending at least 150-300 minutes each week of moderate-intensity exercise is recomended, like brisk walking. Or, you can try a 75-150 minute per week regime with vigorous-intensity physical activity like jogging and running. Both will lower inflammation and allow the natural processes of your body to work optimally.

Avoid alcohol

As mentioned above, alcohol is a harmful substance that can decrease the efficiency of your body's natural ability to detoxify itself. Yes, most of the alcohol you drink will be metabolized by the liver. However, it will also release acetaldehyde, which is a toxin. But the liver will convert the acetaldehyde into acetate, which is then removed from the body.

While it is okay if you drink the recommended glasses of alcohol (two for men and one for women), it is always better to avoid alcohol. Apart from weakening your body's natural detoxification system, it will affect other aspects of your health like the immune system, cholesterol, etc.

Avoiding alcohol does not have to be difficult. Of course, you may find yourself struggling with some withdrawal symptoms. While the list of these symptoms may sound severe, it is not that difficult. Research has found that people can avoid drinking alcohol with little or no side effects. Alternatively, you can also try to not visit alcohol shops. As long as you keep your alcohol intake under the recommended amount, you should be good.

Chapter 6

How to naturally reverse diabetes and lower your blood pressure

D iabetes can strike any person from all walks of life. Today, there are more than 422 million people around the world that have been diagnosed with diabetes, with approximately 30 million in American alone. Without careful and ongoing management, it can lead to serious complications like heart diseases and stroke.

What is diabetes?

Diabetes is a serious health condition that causes excess blood sugar levels. It is normally caused when the body is unable to use its own insulin, a hormone secreted by the pancreas. Insulin is the key to open the cells, which will allow glucose (sugar) from the food you eat to enter. Next, this glucose will be used by the body for energy.

When it comes to diabetes, there are a lot of things that can go wrong and cause a problem. The most common types of diabetes are Type-1 and Type-2 diabetes. However, there are also some other forms of diabetes, like gestational diabetes, that occur during pregnancy.

Role of insulin in diabetes

The human body is made up of millions of cells. When you drink or eat, the food is broken down into glucose, which is transported to various parts of the body via the bloodstream and provides the energy that your body needs for different activities.

The amount of glucose you have in your bloodstream is regulated by the insulin hormone, which is released by the pancreas. When the glucose rises to a certain level, the pancreas will release insulin to push the glucose into the cells and drop the blood glucose levels.

What are the different types of diabetes?

Some different types of diabetes are:

Type-1 diabetes

Also known as juvenile diabetes, Type-1 diabetes is the most severe type of disease. Approximately 5% of people around the world suffer from Type-1 diabetes, or also known as insulin-dependent diabetes. This type of diabetes is known as juvenile diabetes because it mostly develops in children and teenagers. However, it occurs in people of all age groups.

When you suffer from Type-1 diabetes, the immune system of your body will attack the insulin-producing islet cells that are secreted from the pancreas. The islet cells can sense the glucose level in your blood and will subsequently produce the right amount of insulin to bring your sugar levels back to normal. The attack on the body's own cells is called autoimmune disease; experts are not very sure why such an attack takes place.

In Type-1 diabetes, the person can no longer produce their own supply of insulin once the insulin-producing cells are destroyed. Without insulin, your cells cannot open up to allow the glucose from the food you eat. Hence, the sugar stays in the blood and starts accumulating. As a result, the cells in your body will start to starve. If left unattended, the high sugar levels in your blood can damage your heart, nerves, kidneys, and eyes; eventually, it may even lead to coma and death.

Treating Type-1 diabetes

Type-1 diabetes can be treated by injecting insulin externally. This insulin from outside will now help your cells absorb glucose. However, the challenge of this method is knowing the exact amount of insulin you need to take. The amount will depend on several factors like

- General and emotional health
- Stress
- Exercise
- Food

The above-mentioned factors can change daily, which can make deciding the insulin dose a very delicate balancing act. If you end up taking more than needed, it can lower your blood sugar level (known as hypoglycemia); this can be life-threatening.

On the other hand, taking less-than-required insulin will raise your blood sugar level. When this happens, your cells will not be getting the glucose or energy they require. This condition is known as hyperglycemia and can also lead to life-threatening complications.

Today, there are many types of diabetes devices that can help people manage their blood sugar levels accurately.

Type-2 diabetes

Another common type of diabetes is Type-2 diabetes, or also known as non-insulin-dependent diabetes. Approximately, 90% of people suffer from Type-2 diabetes. While it usually develops after the age of 35-years (thereby the name adult-onset diabetes), it may also be seen in younger people.

In Type-2 diabetes, people are able to produce some insulin. However, this amount is not enough. Normally, this insulin will open the body's cells to allow glucose to enter. However, the cells will not open at times; this is known as insulin resistance and mostly occurs in people that are overweight and lead a sedentary lifestyle.

Gestational diabetes

Gestational diabetes is a diabetic condition that occurs in women, especially when they are pregnant. In most cases, this type of diabetes will disappear once the baby is born. However, there also have been cases where women suffering from gestational diabetes will develop Type-2 diabetes later in life. At times, diabetes that is diagnosed during pregnancy actually turns out to be Type-2 diabetes.

How do you manage diabetes?

At the moment, diabetes cannot be cured. However, it can be controlled and managed. The goals of managing diabetes are:

- Slow, or possibly prevent, the development of health problems related to diabetes
- Controlling your blood pressure; ideally, it should not get over 130/80
- Maintaining triglyceride (lipid) and blood cholesterol levels as normal as possible by avoiding processed starches and sugars and by reducing cholesterol and saturated fat
- Keeping your blood sugar levels as normal as possible by balancing your food intake, physical activity, and certain medications

You hold the key to managing your diabetes by:

- Keeping and maintaining your appointments with your health care providers and getting your laboratory tests done as ordered by your physician or doctor
- Monitoring your blood pressure and blood sugar levels at home
- Taking your medicines according to the described prescription by following the guidelines on when and how to take it
- Working out and exercising daily
- Planning what you eat and following a balanced meal diet

How common is diabetes?

Overall, Type-2 diabetes is more common than Type-1 diabetes. According to studies, more than 34.2 million people living in America were living with diabetes (diagnosed and undiagnosed) in 2018; this number is roughly one out of ten people. On the other hand, about 90% of people suffer from Type-2 diabetes.

Additionally, the percentage of people that suffer from diabetes increases with age. Among all the people that have diabetes, about 26% of them are above the age of 65-years. Men and women are equally prone to getting diabetes. However, the prevalence rate will depend on ethnicities and races. For instance, Mexican Americans, Alaskan Natives, and American Indians are more prone to diabetes. In general, Hispanic and Black populations have higher rates of diabetes than non-Hispanic Asians and non-Hispanic whites.

Additionally, prevalence rates are higher for Hispanic Americans of Puerto Rican or Mexican descent than those of Cuban or South or Central American descent. Among the non-Hispanic Asian population, people with Asian Indian ancestry are more susceptible to diabetes than those with Filipino or Chinese ancestry.

Symptoms of diabetes

The following symptoms of diabetes are very typical; however, some people may have symptoms that may go unnoticed. Hence, it is important that you know the common symptoms of all types of diabetes.

Symptoms of Type-1 diabetes

Some common Type-1 diabetes symptoms include:

Unusual thirst

One of the most common symptoms of Type-1 diabetes is an unusual thirst. This condition causes the kindest to eliminate excess sugar in the blood by removing more water. The water is eliminated from the body via urination, which causes dehydration; thereby, you end up drinking more water.

Weight loss

People suffering from Type-1 diabetes unintentionally lose a significant amount of weight and also increase their appetite. This is because the sugar levels in the blood remain high and the body starts to metabolize the fat for energy. Glucose metabolism gets disrupted and causes the person to feel drowsy and lazy for an extended period. The weight loss is also caused by excessive urination because the calories exit the body in the urine.

Skin problems

The disruption of glucose metabolism also causes changes in the skin condition of Type-1 diabetes. Patients with Type-1 diabetes are more prone to fungal infections and bacterial infections. The blood may not even circulate in the skin properly. Most patients suffer from fungal infections commonly caused by the yeast Candida albicans. These infections can cause a variety of diseases like ringworm, jock itch, vaginal yeast infection in women, athlete's foot, and diaper rash in babies.

Ketoacidosis symptoms

Because the cells are deprived of the sugar they need, they will start burning fat for energy. Eventually, this leads to increased ketone levels in the blood. These acids can change the pH level of the blood and trigger a life-threatening coma. Symptoms of diabetic ketoacidosis include confusion, loss of appetite, rapid breathing, flushed or dry skin, and drowsiness, apart from the other typical symptoms of diabetes. This is a medical emergency and needs to be treated in a hospital setting quickly.

Other symptoms

Type-1 diabetes, when left untreated, can cause many other serious symptoms like diabetic coma, dry mouth, fruity breath, fatigue, loss of consciousness, tingling or numbness in the extremities (especially in the feet), and blurry visions. Diabetic coma and loss of consciousness are considered medical emergencies.

Symptoms of Type-2 diabetes

Some early symptoms of Type-2 diabetes include:

Repeated urination

If you have high sugar levels in your blood, your kidneys will attempt to eliminate the extra sugar content by filtering it out of the bloodstream. This causes the person to urinate more than usual, especially at night.

Increased thirst

With frequent urination comes increased thirst. When the body is removing the excess sugar from the body, it also causes the body to lose additional water. Over time, this can cause dehydration and will make you feel thirstier than usual.

Increased hunger

People with diabetes are often not able to absorb all the nutrients from the food they consume. When the body breaks down the food, it gets converted into a simple sugar known as glucose; the body then uses the glucose as fuel. People suffering from Type-2 diabetes do not have enough glucose the moves from the bloodstream into the body's cells. As a result, they are constantly hungry, no matter how recently they have eaten.

Blurry vision

Too much sugar in the blood could cause damage to the blood vessels of the eyes, thereby resulting in blurry vision. The blurriness can occur in one or both eyes and may come and go. If this symptom is left untreated for long, the damage to these blood vessels becomes more severe and could eventually lead to permanent blindness.

Pain, numbness, or a tingling sensation in the feet and hands

The high blood sugar level can disrupt blood circulation and can damage the nerves. In the case of Type-2 diabetes, this can lead to numbness, a tingling sensation, or pain in the feet and hands. This condition, also known as neuropathy, gets worse if left untreated and often leads to more serious complications.

Symptoms of Gestational diabetes

The symptoms of gestational diabetes are the same as Type-1 and Type-2 diabetes. The difference is that these symptoms occur mostly between the 24th and 28th week of pregnancy. The symptoms include:

- Weight loss
- Blurred vision
- Excess hunger/thirst
- Frequent urination

What is high blood pressure?

By definition, high blood pressure, or also known as hypertension, occurs when blood starts pushing against the walls of the blood vessels with more force.

How do blood pressure and circulatory system work?

To function normally and survive, the organs and the tissues require oxygenated blood, which is carried by the circulatory system throughout the body. When the heart beats, the pressure is created that pushes the blood through the blood vessels – namely, the arteries, the veins, and the capillaries. This pressure is known as blood pressure.

There are two types of forces at play here – the first force is known as systolic pressure and occurs when blood is being pumped out of the heart and into the arteries, which are a part of the circulatory system. Diastolic pressure is the second force that is created when the heart is resting between the rhythmic beats.

Causes of high blood pressure

There are two types of high blood pressure or hypertension. Both types have different causes:

Primary hypertension

Also known as essential hypertension, this type of hypertension can develop over time with no identifiable cause. This is the most common type of blood pressure.

According to experts, it is still unclear why blood pressure increases slowly. There may be a combination of several factors playing a role, some of which include:

- **Genes**

Some people are genetically predisposed to high blood pressure. This may be because of genetic abnormalities inherited from parents or gene mutation.

- **Physical changes**

When your body goes through changes, you will start experiencing issues throughout your body. One of these issues is hypertension. For instance, it is often said that old age brings about changes to the normal functioning of the kidneys, which can change the natural balance of fluids and salts in the body. This results in increased blood pressure.

- **Environment**

Over time, unhealthy lifestyle choices can lead to certain lifestyle choices like poor diet and lack of physical activities, which takes a toll on the body. Bad lifestyle choices can lead to weight problems. Being obese or overweight can also contribute towards hypertension.

Secondary hypertension

Secondary hypertension can occur fast and can become more severe than primary hypertension. Some factors that can cause secondary hypertension include:

- Some types of endocrine tumors
- Problems in the adrenal gland
- Chronic abuse of alcohol
- Use of illegal drugs
- Side effects of medications
- Problems with the thyroid
- Congenital heart defects
- Obstructive sleep apnea
- Kidney diseases

How to diagnose high blood pressure?

Diagnosing high blood pressure is very easy. All you need to do is take a blood pressure reading. Most doctors will check your blood pressure as part of a routine visit. If you do not receive a blood pressure reading during your appointment, you can simply request one.

If your blood pressure is more than the safe level, the doctor will request more readings in the span of the next few days or weeks. A diagnosis for hypertension is rarely given only after the first reading. The doctor will take more readings to determine whether it is evidence of a potentially sustained problem. This is because increased blood pressure also depends on the environment, like the stress you feel in an office. Also, blood pressure can change throughout the day.

If your blood pressure still remains high, the doctor will conduct more tests like:

- Ultrasound of the kidneys or heart
- Test the electrical activity of your heart
- Blood tests and cholesterol screening
- Urine test

Understanding high blood pressure readings

There are two numbers that are typically used to measure blood pressure:

Systolic pressure

This is the top (or first) number that indicates the pressure in the arteries when the heart is beating to pump out blood.

Diastolic pressure

This is the bottom (or second) number that measures the pressure of your arteries when the heart is resting between the beats.

For adults, there are five types of blood pressure readings:

Healthy

By default, healthy blood pressure should not be more than 120/80 mm Hg (millimeters of mercury). This means your blood pressure is exactly how it should be.

Elevated

Blood pressure can be said as elevated if the systolic number is between 120 and 129 mm Hg and the diastolic number is lower than 80mm. Doctors would not normally treat elevated blood pressure with medication; instead, they would encourage lifestyle changes to lower the numbers.

Stage 1 hypertension

This stage of hypertension usually has the systolic number between 130 and 139 mm Hg and the diastolic number at or above 90 mm Hg.

Hypertensive crisis

The hypertensive crisis requires medical attention. The systolic number is well above 180 mm Hg and the diastolic number is more than 120 mm Hg. Some of its symptoms include visual changes, shortness of breath, headache, and pain when the blood pressure is high.

Also, heed that the blood pressure readings for children and teenagers are different. To monitor their blood pressure, ask the doctor for the healthy range.

How common is high blood pressure?

Many people all over the World suffer from high blood pressure. It has been estimated that approximately 18% of adult men and 13% of women suffer from high blood pressure or hypertension; however, they are not getting the treatment done. In almost 95% of the cases, while there are many reasons for increasing blood pressure, lifestyle is the most common one, according to experts.

Additionally, people of Afro-Caribbean descent and South Asian (India, Bangladesh, and Pakistan) origin are more prone to developing high blood pressure than other ethnic groups; the reason is not fully understood, as for now.

Symptoms of high blood pressure

If you are looking for a list of signs and symptoms of high blood pressure (hypertension), you will not find them. One reason is that there are none.

- **Myth**: People with high blood pressure experience symptoms like facial flushing, difficulty sleeping, sweating, and nervousness.
- **Truth**: High blood pressure is notoriously known as the 'silent killer' because it is largely symptomless. If you ignore your blood pressure because you think you will notice a certain sign or symptom of the problem, you are taking a heavy risk on your life.

Some expert recommendations include:

- You should never attempt to self-diagnose. Always opt for clinical diagnosis under a healthcare professional.
- It is important for you to know your blood pressure numbers and make the necessary changes to your lifestyle to protect your health.

High blood pressure does not cause nosebleeds or headaches

According to experts, high blood pressure does not cause nosebleeds or headaches. However, a case of a hypertensive crisis (mentioned above) falls under medical emergency; the blood pressure during a hypertensive crisis is over 180/120 mm Hg. Having an unusually high blood pressure will cause you to suffer from nosebleeds and headaches; if you start feeling unwell, you should wait for some minutes and take a brief rest. If your blood pressure remains the same, call a doctor immediately.

If you are experiencing severe nosebleeds, headaches, and feeling unwell, get in touch with your doctor as they could be symptoms of other health diseases.

Inconclusively-related symptoms

There is a wide range of symptoms that might be related to, but not always caused by, blood pressure, like:

Dizziness

In most cases, dizziness can be a side effect of medications for high blood pressure. However, it is not caused by high blood pressure. However, you should not ignore dizziness, especially if the onset is immediate. Sudden dizziness, trouble walking, and loss of coordination or balance are warning signs of a stroke. Coincidentally, high blood pressure is the leading risk factor for a stroke.

Facial flushing

Facial flushing takes place when the blood vessels in your face start to dilate. It can either be a response to certain triggers like skin-care products, hot drinks, wind, spicy foods, cold weather, and sun exposure or can occur unpredictably. Facial flushing also happens due to exercise, alcohol consumption, exposure to cold or hot water, and emotional stress – all of which can temporarily increase your blood pressure. While the flushing does take place when your blood pressure is higher than normal, it is definitely not a cause of hypertension.

Blood spots in the eyes

Subconjunctival hemorrhage, or blood spots in the eyes, is more common in people with high blood pressure and diabetes. However, it does not mean that either of the conditions is responsible for the blood spots. The spots in the eyes do not relate to high blood pressure in any way. However, it is recommended that you get in touch with an ophthalmologist as soon as possible. The eye doctor will then be able to detect the damage to the optic nerve that is caused by high blood pressure if left unchecked.

Diet

Figuring out the best foods you need to eat when you are diabetic can be tough. This is mostly because your goal is all about controlling your blood sugar levels. However, it is just as important to eat foods that help you prevent complications like heart problems. Here are the types of foods that people living with diabetes can eat:

Low glycemic index foods

Eating low-glycemic index foods is a tool that will help keep your diabetes under control. The glycemic index is a type of food rating system to measure the number of carbohydrates. It will help you understand how fast food will raise your blood sugar level. This way, you will only focus on foods that do not raise your blood sugar so fast.

It is recommended that you eat low-glycemic foods with diets planned for diabetes, like carbohydrate counting. Counting the number of carbs you consume will give you an estimated idea of how much carbohydrates you consume.

Foods rich in chromium and magnesium

Chromium is a trace element that is found in almost all types of foods. According to research, chromium has been known to reduce insulin resistance. Additionally, the element will also enhance the effects of insulin and improve blood sugar levels.

A deficiency of magnesium in your diet can lead to Type-1 and Type-2 diabetes. This is because low levels of magnesium are often associated with insulin resistance. People with insulin sensitivity also lose magnesium via urination.

Apple cider vinegar

Apple cider vinegar is known to have a lot of health benefits. While it may contain apples, the fruit sugar is fermented and converted into acetic acid. As a result, a single teaspoon will not contain more than a gram of carbs.

According to studies, it has been found that apple cider adds a lot of beneficial effects on lowering HbA1c and blood sugar levels. In fact, the blood sugar levels may fall as much as 20% when consumed with meals that contain carbs.

Berberine

Berberine is a chemical that is found in many plants like tree turmeric, Phellodendron, Oregon grape, greater celandine, goldthread, and the European barberry. This chemical is commonly taken by people suffering from high blood pressure, high cholesterol levels, and diabetes.

Berberine helps the heart to beat more robustly, which helps people with some types of heart conditions. Berberine also regulates how the body uses the blood sugar content. This is especially helpful for people suffering from diabetes. Additionally, the chemical is also used for other purposes like treating liver diseases and burns.

Fenugreek seeds

Scientifically known as Trigonellafoenumgraecum, fenugreek seeds are high in soluble fiber, which will help lower blood sugar levels by absorbing carbohydrates and slowing down the digestion process. This has been proven to be one of the most effective methods of treating diabetics.

Additional research has proved that fenugreek seed will reduce the fasting blood sugar levels in insulin-dependent (Type-1) diabetics. This means that it can improve glucose tolerance as well.

Whole wheat or pumpernickel bread

Bread is a popular food all around the world. However, bread contains a high amount of carbohydrates, which is not good news for diabetic people. However, there are some types of bread that contain low levels of carbs.

Most of these bread variations are homemade and available easily at farmers' markets. They are local and have higher fiber content with minimum sugar. They are also less likely processed than the ones you see at grocery stores. Hence, you do not have to eliminate bread from your diet. You simply need to switch to whole wheat or pumpernickel bread.

Fruits

Eating fruits is one of the best ways to maintain good health. However, most fruits contain sugar, which has raised questions on whether they are suitable for diabetics. According to research, any fruit is fine to eat, even for a person with diabetes, as long as the person is not allergic to a particular fruit.

Additional studies have shown that higher fruit intake will drastically lower the risk of diabetes, especially Type-2 diabetes. It is suggested that diabetics eat fruits in their natural form and avoid processed or canned fruit products.

Sweet potatoes and yams

In the past few years, sweet potatoes and yams have garnered the attention of people suffering from diabetes, mostly thanks to their low glycemic index rating. As mentioned previously, foods that are ranked higher in the GI (glycemic index) scale may cause your blood sugar levels to increase faster. Sweet potatoes are ranked much lower than white potatoes on the GI scale.

Additionally, they are also a great source of protein that will help you feel fuller and promoting weight loss, apart from increasing insulin sensitivity.

Oatmeal and oat bran

Adding oatmeal and oat bran to your diet will do wonders for your diabetic condition. It will help regulate your blood sugar levels, thanks to its low glycemic index and high fiber content. The soluble fiber content and low cholesterol also make it a perfect choice for maintaining perfect heart health.

Proper consumption of oatmeal and oat bran will reduce your need for insulin injections, especially if eaten with other breakfast foods that are rich in carbohydrates. Lastly, it is something that you can cook quickly.

Nuts

Nuts are nutritious and delicious. All types of nuts are low in net carb and contain fiber, although some varieties have more than others. For instance, one ounce of almonds contains 2.6 grams of digestible carbs and cashews have 7.7 grams.

It has been studied on various types of nuts that regular consumption will lower blood sugar levels and reduce inflammation. Nuts are also known to improve heart conditions in diabetic people. Additional research also blood glucose levels in people with diabetes.

Legumes

According to studies, it has been proven that people that eat legumes like lentils, peas, and beans regularly are less prone to developing Type-2 diabetes. Additionally, legumes can also help people suffering from Type-2 diabetes manage their blood sugar content.

Legumes are known to reduce the risk or manage Type-2 diabetes because they are rich in nutrients and low on the glycemic index rating. Hence, the food will improve gain more control on the blood glucose level. Eating legumes is an important part of the diet for diabetic patients who are at a greater risk of developing heart diseases and/or being overweight.

Cold-water fish

Some experts consider cold-water fish, or fatty fishes, to be one of the healthiest types of foods on earth. Fishes like mackerel, anchovies, herring, sardines, and salmon are the best sources of omega-3 fatty acids like EPA and DHA, which are greatly beneficial for heart health.

For diabetic people, getting enough of these fats is very important to decrease the risk for a stroke or other heart diseases. EPA and DHA will protect the cells that line the blood vessels, thereby reducing the chances of inflammation and further improving the functioning of the arteries.

Yogurt

Yogurt, especially Greek yogurt, is a great dairy product for diabetic people. According to research, it has been concluded that eating certain dairy products like yogurt will improve the sugar levels in your blood and also reduce the risk of heart diseases, partly thanks to the probiotics that it contains.

Studies have also indicated that yogurt consumption may be associated with insulin resistance and lower levels of blood glucose. Additionally, a long-term study has proved that people eating yogurt daily have an 18% lower risk of developing diabetes, particularly Type-2 diabetes.

10 natural herbs for high blood pressure

Bacopamonnieri

Also known as the thyme-leaved Graciela, water hyssop, or Brahmi, the Bacopamonnieri is an ancient medicine that is mostly used in Ayurvedic treatments for a wide range of treatments. It mostly grows in tropical and wet environments and can thrive underwater as well.

According to research, it has been found that Bacopamonnieri may keep your blood pressure under a healthy range. It is known to reduce systolic and diastolic pressure by releasing nitric oxide, which dilates the blood vessels. While human trials are yet to be done, Bacopamonnieri has been found to lower blood pressure in rats.

Basil

Basil is a flavorful herb that is often used in different types of foods. However, it is also rich in various powerful compounds that can reduce blood pressure. According to research, basil contains eugenol, which is linked to lowered blood pressure.

Additional studies have concluded that eugenol acts as a natural calcium channel blocker to reduce blood pressure. Calcium channel blockers prevent calcium from entering the arterial cells and the heart, thereby allowing the blood vessels to relax.

Cardamom

According to experts, cardamom is particularly helpful for people suffering from high blood pressure. Medical studies and clinical trials have found that three grams of cardamom will significantly bring down blood pressure within the normal range.

It has also be found that the spice promotes a diuretic effect, which lowers blood pressure; this is because water that builds up in your body, especially around the heart, is flushed out via urination. Its antioxidant properties also play a role in lowering blood pressure.

Celery seeds

It is no secret that celery seeds are great for your health. However, celery seeds are most well-known for improving blood pressure in humans. Celery seeds contain phytochemicals known as phthalides, or also known as NBP. It is known to relax the walls of the artery to reduce blood pressure and increase the flow of blood.

Apart from the seeds, you can also consume celery stalk, which contains potassium, magnesium, and fiber; all these nutrients will help regulate and maintain your blood pressure.

Chinese cat's claw

More popularly known as Chotoko or Gou-Teng, the Chinese cat's claw is an ancient medicine that has been used in ancient China for treating a wide range of ailments. Of course, it does not literally mean a cat's claws. It is a plant that contains several compounds like nitric oxide and hirsute, which reduce blood pressure by acting as natural calcium channel blockers.

Chinese cat's claw also contains other nutrients that stimulate the production of nitric oxide in the blood vessels, which will relax and dilate the vessels. The plant can be found easily in online stores or select health stores.

Cinnamon

According to recent studies, it has been found that cinnamon has a focused effect on blood sugar levels. While the mechanism is yet to be determined, it has been reported that cinnamon provides some benefits for people who are trying to regulate blood sugar levels and control diabetes.

Additionally, cinnamon is also linked to lowering blood sugar levels in the body. While studies are still being conducted, initial tests have proven this theory to be right for now. More research will be required to fully understand the benefits of cinnamon on a person suffering from high blood pressure.

Garlic

The health benefits of garlic have been known and exploited for ages. It is a natural antifungal and antibiotic food that contains allicin, which is linked to several health benefits.

According to studies, it has been found that garlic increases the production of nitric acid in the body, which functions as natural calcium channel blockers as well as helps the blood vessels and muscles relax. All these changes also contribute to reducing hypertension. Additional research concludes that allicin also reduces systolic and diastolic blood pressure, especially in hypertensive individuals.

Ginger

Ginger is one of the most versatile ingredients that are often used in alternative medicine. The herb is known for its medicinal properties and is mostly linked with improving the health of the heart, including blood pressure, cholesterol levels, and circulation.

Studies have concluded that ginger will significantly reduce blood pressure in more than one way. First, it acts as a natural ACE inhibitor and calcium channel blocker, both of which are types of medication for blood pressure. Ginger will also lower the risk of developing high blood pressure.

Parsley

A common flowering plant from the Mediterranean, parsley has been used in treating several types of heart ailments like inflammatory diseases, allergies, and high blood pressure. It is filled with nutrients that improve the health of the heart and the blood vessels.

Rich in iron, parsley improves the RBC count in the blood, which is important to maintain a good heart. The carotenoid in it also helps minimize the risk of high blood pressure and chronic inflammation. By reducing the risk of high blood pressure, parsley also promotes kidney health.

Thyme

Thyme is an appetizing herb that contains a lot of compounds that are good for your health. According to studies, rosmarinic acid is one of those compounds that has been linked with reducing blood sugar levels and reduce inflammation. It also promotes blood flow and is known to regulate blood pressure.

Studies have also concluded that rosamrinic acid also inhibits the ACE (angiotensin-converting enzyme) to reduce systolic pressure; ACE is a molecule that is notoriously known to raise blood pressure by narrowing the blood vessels.

Conclusion

We now understand how our diet plays an important role in regulating several aspects of our body like detoxification, natural cleansing, diabetes, and blood pressure. Toxins in the body can lead to a lot of health complications like heart diseases, stroke, cancer, and diabetes; however, if you manage the food that you eat, you will avoid such health risks and lose some weight in the process.

While the body is made to eliminate toxic materials naturally, there are some that cannot be removed just as easily. As mentioned above, arsenic is one such compound that can cause potential harm or even death.

An alkaline diet is the best solution for the problem. As we have mentioned previously, a simple alkaline diet will improve your physical and mental well-being by ensuring that your blood pH level is constant. Of course, the fluctuation of this pH level would cause the functioning of several types of cells and will lead to health problems.

We also talked about detoxification. This can go hand-in-hand with your alkaline diet. When you are going through a detoxification process, you will consume less harmful substances and eliminate the ones in your body easily. The body keeps producing toxic by-products like lactic acid that are particularly bad for your health.

Thankfully, detoxification is just about how strong you are to give up processed foods and products that produce the most toxins like dairy, gluten, eggs, and red meat. Most detox programs focus on foods that are grown naturally like gluten-free grains, nuts, seeds, lean proteins, and vegetables. Of course, you can also opt for fasting; however, studies have concluded that fasting can be risky for the human body. Therefore, most medical experts would not recommend fasting and instead encourage specific types of diets like an alkaline diet.

All these aspects are quite important, especially when it comes to the health of your liver. One of the most important liver functions is to remove toxins from your body. If it becomes toxic, it can have a very bad effect on your body. In most cases, a toxic liver is caused by consuming alcohol, drugs, chemicals, and certain nutritional supplements.

Apart from implementing an alkaline diet into your routine by opting for a detox, cleansing your liver is also possible. All you need to do are follow certain steps mentioned in Chapter 3. There are also many other home remedies you can try, like incorporating turmeric or milk thistle into your diet.

Lastly, we also talked about high blood pressure and diabetes, both conditions that are prevalent in society today. Of course, your genes may also be blamed for it. However, it is important that you minimize external habits that can lead to these conditions. It is a fact that such health problems will not allow you to live peacefully and will cause a lot of inconveniences.

CPSIA information can be obtained
at www.ICGtesting.com
Printed in the USA
BVHW091941120521
607126BV00014B/2472